Table Of Contents

Chapter 1: The Science Behind Telomerase Activation: Exploring the Effects of Ashwagandha

Introduction to Telomeres and Telomerase

In this subchapter, we will delve into the fascinating world of telomeres and telomerase, and explore their connection to the aging process. Whether you are a curious individual or someone seeking to unlock the secrets of youthful longevity, this chapter will provide you with valuable insights into the science behind telomerase activation and the remarkable effects of Ashwagandha.

Telomeres are the protective caps at the ends of our chromosomes. Think of them as the plastic tips on shoelaces that prevent fraying – they play a crucial role in maintaining the stability and integrity of our DNA. However, as we age, our telomeres naturally shorten and lose their ability to protect our genetic material effectively. This process has been linked to the development of age-related diseases and the overall decline in our health.

Fortunately, telomerase, an enzyme found in our bodies, has the power to counteract telomere shortening. Telomerase works by adding DNA sequences to the ends of our telomeres, effectively lengthening them and maintaining their function. The activation of telomerase has been shown to slow down the aging process, promote cellular rejuvenation, and extend the lifespan of various organisms.

One potent natural compound that has gained significant attention in the field of telomere research is Ashwagandha. This ancient herb, long revered in Ayurvedic medicine, has been found to possess remarkable telomerase activation properties. Studies have shown that Ashwagandha root extract can increase telomerase activity, leading to the preservation of telomere length and potentially reversing the aging process.

In this book, we will guide you through the science behind telomerase activation and the effects of Ashwagandha on telomeres. We will explore how Ashwagandha can unlock the fountain of youth by activating telomeres, allowing you to turn back the biological clock and experience youthful longevity. We will provide you with a step-by-step guide to the Ashwagandha telomere protocol, enabling you to harness the power of this incredible herb to reverse aging and rejuvenate your body.

Whether you are seeking to understand the revolutionary effects of Ashwagandha on aging or looking for practical ways to incorporate it into your daily life, this subchapter will provide you with the knowledge and tools you need. Get ready to embark on a journey of discovery as we uncover the secrets of telomeres, telomerase, and the transformative potential of Ashwagandha for a youthful and vibrant future.

The Role of Telomeres in Aging

Telomeres, the protective caps at the ends of our chromosomes, play a crucial role in the aging process. As we age, these telomeres naturally shorten and become frayed, leading to cellular dysfunction and ultimately contributing to the onset of age-related diseases. However, recent scientific advancements have shed light on the potential of telomerase activation to reverse this process and promote youthful longevity. In this subchapter, we will explore the role of telomeres in aging and how the powerful herb Ashwagandha can be used to activate telomeres and unlock the fountain of youth.

Telomeres act as the biological clock of our cells, determining their lifespan. Each time a cell divides, its telomeres shorten, and once they reach a critical length, the cell can no longer divide and becomes senescent or dies. This progressive shortening of telomeres is a natural part of aging, but various environmental factors, such as stress, poor nutrition, and exposure to toxins, can accelerate this process.

The groundbreaking discovery of telomerase, an enzyme that can lengthen telomeres, has opened up new possibilities for combating aging. Telomerase activation has been shown to rejuvenate cells, improve their function, and potentially slow down the aging process. This is where Ashwagandha, a powerful adaptogenic herb, comes into play.

Ashwagandha has been used for centuries in traditional Ayurvedic medicine for its rejuvenating and anti-aging properties. Recent scientific studies have shown that Ashwagandha can stimulate telomerase activity, leading to the lengthening of telomeres and the promotion of cellular health. By activating telomeres, Ashwagandha has the potential to turn back the biological clock and reverse the signs of aging.

In this subchapter, we will delve into the science behind telomerase activation and explore the effects of Ashwagandha on telomeres. We will provide a step-by-step guide to using Ashwagandha to activate telomeres and reverse aging. From understanding the mechanisms behind telomerase activation to exploring the revolutionary effects of Ashwagandha on aging, this subchapter aims to unlock the secrets of youthful longevity.

Whether you are interested in the science behind telomerase activation, seeking a guide to reversing aging through telomere activation, or simply looking for ways to improve your overall well-being and promote a youthful you, this subchapter will provide you with the knowledge and tools to harness the power of Ashwagandha and unlock the potential of your telomeres.

Join the anti-aging revolution and discover how Ashwagandha can help you turn back the biological clock for a healthier, more vibrant life.

Understanding Telomerase and its Function

Telomeres have long been associated with the aging process, acting as protective caps on the ends of our chromosomes. As we age, these telomeres naturally shorten, leading to cellular damage and ultimately, the onset of age-related diseases. However, recent scientific breakthroughs have revealed the potential of telomerase and its role in reversing the aging process.

Telomerase is an enzyme that plays a crucial role in maintaining the length and integrity of telomeres. It works by adding repetitive DNA sequences to the ends of chromosomes, effectively preventing them from shortening. This process of telomere elongation is vital for the preservation of cell function and overall health.

In the book "The Telomere Breakthrough: Unleashing Ashwagandha's Potential for Age Reversal," we explore the fascinating science behind telomerase activation and its relationship with the powerful herb, Ashwagandha. Ashwagandha has been used for centuries in Ayurvedic medicine for its rejuvenating properties, and recent research has shown its potential in activating telomerase and extending the lifespan of cells.

Unlocking the Fountain of Youth: A Guide to Activating Telomeres with Ashwagandha delves into the mechanisms by which Ashwagandha stimulates telomerase activity. By increasing telomerase levels, Ashwagandha helps to maintain the length of telomeres and protect against cellular aging and damage.

Furthermore, Ashwagandha and Longevity: How to Reverse Aging through Telomere Activation explores the potential of Ashwagandha in reversing the aging process. By activating telomeres, Ashwagandha may hold the key to youthful longevity and improved healthspan.

The Telomere Solution: Using Ashwagandha to Turn Back the Biological Clock provides practical insights into incorporating

Ashwagandha into your daily routine to support telomere health. This step-by-step guide outlines the recommended dosage, best practices, and potential side effects to ensure safe and effective telomere activation.

In The Ashwagandha Telomere Protocol: A Step-by-Step Guide to Reversing Aging, we present a comprehensive protocol for utilizing Ashwagandha to activate telomeres and reverse the effects of aging. This protocol covers diet, exercise, and lifestyle changes that can further enhance the benefits of Ashwagandha supplementation.

Telomeres Unleashed: The Revolutionary Effects of Ashwagandha on Aging explores the groundbreaking research on Ashwagandha's effects on telomeres and aging. By understanding the science behind this revolutionary herb, we can unlock its potential for a youthful and vibrant life.

In summary, this subchapter aims to provide a comprehensive understanding of telomerase and its function in the context of aging. By exploring the effects of Ashwagandha on telomere activation, we hope to empower everyone to take control of their own aging process and unlock the secrets to a youthful and vibrant life.

Telomerase Activation and its Potential Benefits

Telomerase Activation and its Potential Benefits

Telomeres, the protective caps at the end of our chromosomes, play a crucial role in the aging process. As we age, these telomeres naturally shorten, leading to cellular damage and the onset of aging-related diseases. However, recent scientific advancements have shed light on an exciting potential solution - telomerase activation. In this subchapter, we will explore the concept of telomerase activation and its potential benefits, specifically focusing on the effects of Ashwagandha, a powerful herb that has shown promising results in this field.

Telomerase is an enzyme responsible for maintaining the length of telomeres. By activating telomerase, we can potentially slow down or even reverse the aging process. Ashwagandha, a herb widely used in traditional Ayurvedic medicine, has been found to have telomerase activating properties. Research studies have shown that Ashwagandha can increase telomerase activity, leading to longer and healthier telomeres.

The potential benefits of telomerase activation through Ashwagandha are manifold. Firstly, it can promote cellular rejuvenation, allowing cells to function optimally and delay the onset of age-related diseases. Secondly, it may enhance cognitive function and improve brain health, as studies have shown a correlation between telomere length and cognitive decline. By activating telomerase, Ashwagandha could potentially protect against neurodegenerative disorders such as Alzheimer's disease.

Furthermore, telomerase activation has been linked to increased energy levels and improved immune function. As we age, our immune system weakens, making us more susceptible to infections and diseases. By activating telomerase, Ashwagandha may boost the immune system's ability to defend against pathogens, leading to better overall health and vitality.

It is important to note that while the potential benefits of telomerase activation through Ashwagandha are promising, further research is required to fully understand its mechanisms and long-term effects. Additionally, it is advisable to consult with a healthcare professional before incorporating Ashwagandha or any other supplements into your daily routine.

In conclusion, telomerase activation holds tremendous potential in the field of anti-aging and longevity. Ashwagandha, with its telomerase activating properties, may offer a natural and safe way to slow down the aging process and unlock the fountain of youth. By understanding the science behind telomerase activation and exploring the effects of Ashwagandha, we can potentially harness the power of this ancient herb to reverse aging and enjoy a youthful and vibrant life.

Exploring the Link Between Ashwagandha and Telomeres

In recent years, scientists and researchers have been captivated by the potential of ashwagandha to reverse the effects of aging. One area of particular interest is the link between ashwagandha and telomeres, the protective caps at the ends of our chromosomes that play a crucial role in the aging process.

Telomeres have been likened to the plastic tips at the end of shoelaces – they prevent our DNA from unraveling and protect it from damage. However, as we age, our telomeres naturally shorten, leaving our DNA vulnerable to deterioration and increasing the risk of age-related diseases.

But what if there was a way to slow down this process, to protect our telomeres and potentially even reverse their aging? This is where ashwagandha comes into play.

Ashwagandha, a powerful adaptogenic herb with a rich history in Ayurvedic medicine, has been found to activate an enzyme called telomerase. Telomerase has the ability to lengthen telomeres, effectively slowing down the aging process at a cellular level.

Studies have shown that ashwagandha extract increases telomerase activity, leading to longer telomeres and ultimately healthier cells. This has profound implications for overall health and longevity.

By activating telomerase with ashwagandha, we have the potential to protect our DNA from damage, reduce the risk of age-related diseases such as cancer and heart disease, and even reverse the signs of aging.

But how can we harness the power of ashwagandha to activate telomeres and unlock the fountain of youth? The answer lies in incorporating ashwagandha into our daily routines.

Whether it's in the form of a supplement, a tea, or a powder, ashwagandha can be easily integrated into our diet and lifestyle. By taking ashwagandha regularly, we can support our body's natural ability to activate telomeres and promote healthy aging.

In conclusion, the link between ashwagandha and telomeres holds great promise for those seeking to reverse the effects of aging. By incorporating ashwagandha into our daily routines, we can unlock the potential of this powerful herb and tap into the secrets of youthful longevity.

So why wait? Start your journey towards a more youthful you with ashwagandha and unleash the power of telomeres.

The Science of Ashwagandha's Effects on Telomerase Activation

Ashwagandha, a powerful herb with a long history in Ayurvedic medicine, has gained significant attention in recent years for its potential to reverse aging and promote longevity. One of the key mechanisms behind its anti-aging effects is its ability to activate telomerase, an enzyme that plays a crucial role in maintaining the length and integrity of our telomeres.

Telomeres, the protective caps at the ends of our chromosomes, act as the biological clock of our cells, determining their lifespan and overall health. As we age, our telomeres naturally shorten, leading to cellular aging and increased susceptibility to age-related diseases. However, research has shown that telomerase activation can counteract this process, promoting cellular rejuvenation and extending lifespan.

Studies have demonstrated that ashwagandha can enhance telomerase activity, effectively slowing down telomere shortening and even lengthening them in some cases. This remarkable effect is attributed to the herb's rich array of bioactive compounds, such as withanolides and alkaloids, which possess potent antioxidant and anti-inflammatory properties.

By reducing oxidative stress and chronic inflammation, ashwagandha helps protect telomeres from damage and degradation. Additionally, it stimulates the production of telomerase, promoting the repair and regeneration of telomeres. This dual action of ashwagandha makes it a powerful ally in the fight against aging and age-related disorders.

Furthermore, ashwagandha's telomerase activation properties have been linked to a range of health benefits beyond just anti-aging. It has been found to enhance immune function, improve cognitive performance, boost energy levels, and reduce the risk of chronic diseases such as cardiovascular disease and cancer.

Incorporating ashwagandha into your daily routine can be done through various forms, including supplements, powders, or teas. However, it's important to note that ashwagandha should be used in moderation and under the guidance of a healthcare professional, especially if you have any pre-existing medical conditions or are taking medications.

In conclusion, the science of ashwagandha's effects on telomerase activation offers a promising approach to reversing aging and promoting youthful longevity. By harnessing the power of this ancient herb, we can unlock the fountain of youth and embark on a journey towards a healthier, more vibrant life.

Chapter 2: Unlocking the Fountain of Youth: A Guide to Activating Telomeres with Ashwagandha

The History and Origins of Ashwagandha

Ashwagandha, also known as Withania somnifera, is an ancient herb that has been used for centuries in Ayurvedic medicine. Its name is derived from the Sanskrit words "ashva," meaning horse, and "gandha," meaning smell, as the root of the plant is said to have a strong horse-like odor.

The history of ashwagandha can be traced back to India, where it has been a staple in traditional medicine for over 3,000 years. It is considered one of the most important herbs in Ayurveda, a holistic healing system that aims to balance the mind, body, and spirit.

According to ancient texts, ashwagandha was believed to possess potent rejuvenating and restorative properties. It was often used to enhance vitality, promote longevity, and improve overall health and well-being. In fact, the herb was often referred to as "rasayana," which translates to "that which promotes youthfulness."

The origins of ashwagandha can be found in the arid regions of India, where it thrives in sandy and dry soil. The plant is a member of the nightshade family and features small, yellow flowers and red berries. However, it is the root of the ashwagandha plant that is most prized for its medicinal properties.

Over the years, ashwagandha has gained recognition worldwide for its numerous health benefits. Modern scientific research has revealed that the herb contains a unique blend of bioactive compounds, including alkaloids, steroidal lactones, and withanolides, which contribute to its therapeutic effects.

One of the most intriguing aspects of ashwagandha is its potential to activate telomerase, an enzyme that plays a vital role in maintaining the length of telomeres – the protective caps at the ends of our chromosomes. Telomeres naturally shorten as we age, leading to cellular aging and an increased risk of age-related diseases.

By activating telomerase, ashwagandha may help slow down the aging process and promote longevity. Research has shown that the herb can increase telomerase activity, resulting in longer telomeres and improved cellular health.

In conclusion, the history and origins of ashwagandha can be traced back to ancient India, where it has been used for thousands of years in Ayurvedic medicine. This powerful herb has gained recognition worldwide for its potential to activate telomerase and promote youthfulness. As more research is conducted, ashwagandha's potential for age reversal is becoming increasingly evident, making it a promising ingredient in the quest for a more youthful and healthy life.

Ashwagandha's Traditional Uses for Health and Longevity

Ashwagandha, also known as Withania somnifera or Indian ginseng, is an ancient herb that has been used for centuries in traditional Ayurvedic medicine. In recent years, it has gained significant attention for its potential to promote health and longevity, particularly through its effects on telomeres.

Telomeres are the protective caps at the end of our chromosomes that shorten as we age. When telomeres become too short, cells can no longer divide and function properly, leading to the aging process. However, scientific research has shown that certain compounds, like those found in ashwagandha, can activate an enzyme called telomerase, which can lengthen telomeres and potentially reverse the aging process.

One of the traditional uses of ashwagandha is as an adaptogen, a substance that helps the body adapt to stress and promote overall well-being. By reducing stress levels, ashwagandha can support the health of telomeres and promote longevity.

Another traditional use of ashwagandha is as a rejuvenating tonic for the mind and body. It is believed to enhance mental clarity, improve memory, and increase energy levels. By supporting cognitive function and overall vitality, ashwagandha can contribute to a healthier and more youthful life.

Ashwagandha has also been used traditionally to boost the immune system and improve overall immune function. By enhancing the body's defenses, ashwagandha can help protect against age-related diseases and contribute to a longer, healthier life.

Additionally, ashwagandha is known for its anti-inflammatory properties, which can help reduce the risk of chronic diseases associated with aging. By fighting inflammation, ashwagandha can support a healthier body and potentially extend lifespan.

In conclusion, ashwagandha has a rich history of traditional use for promoting health and longevity. Its adaptogenic properties, rejuvenating effects, immune-boosting abilities, and anti-inflammatory properties all contribute to its potential to reverse the aging process by activating telomeres. By incorporating ashwagandha into your daily routine, you can harness its power and unlock the secrets to a more youthful and vibrant life.

Disclaimer: The content provided here is for informational purposes only and is not intended as medical advice. Always consult with a qualified healthcare professional before starting any new supplementation or treatment regimen.

The Active Compounds in Ashwagandha and their Effects on Telomeres

Ashwagandha, known by its scientific name Withania somnifera, is a powerful herb that has been used for centuries in traditional Ayurvedic medicine. In recent years, it has gained significant attention in the field of anti-aging research, specifically in relation to its effects on telomeres.

Telomeres are the protective caps at the ends of our chromosomes that shorten as we age. When telomeres become too short, cells can no longer divide and function properly, leading to the aging process and an increased risk of age-related diseases. Therefore, finding ways to maintain or even lengthen telomeres is of great interest to scientists and individuals seeking to slow down or reverse the aging process.

Ashwagandha contains several active compounds that have been found to have positive effects on telomeres. One of these compounds is called withaferin A, which has been shown to activate an enzyme called telomerase. Telomerase is responsible for maintaining the length of telomeres by adding DNA sequences to their ends. By activating telomerase, withaferin A can potentially help to preserve telomere length and delay the aging process.

Additionally, ashwagandha is rich in antioxidants, such as flavonoids and phenolic compounds, which can help to reduce oxidative stress and inflammation in the body. Oxidative stress and inflammation are known to accelerate telomere shortening, so by reducing these factors, ashwagandha may indirectly help to maintain telomere length.

Furthermore, studies have shown that ashwagandha has a positive impact on stress and cortisol levels. Chronic stress has been linked to accelerated telomere shortening and premature aging. Ashwagandha's ability to reduce stress and cortisol levels may therefore have a protective effect on telomeres and contribute to a more youthful and healthy aging process.

In conclusion, ashwagandha contains active compounds, such as withaferin A, antioxidants, and stress-reducing properties, that have the potential to positively impact telomeres.

By activating telomerase, reducing oxidative stress and inflammation, and managing stress levels, ashwagandha may contribute to the maintenance or even lengthening of telomeres, thus promoting a more youthful and healthy aging process.

Incorporating ashwagandha into your daily routine may be a promising strategy for those interested in unlocking the fountain of youth and enhancing longevity.

The Mechanisms of Action for Ashwagandha in Telomere Activation

Ashwagandha, a powerful herb derived from the Withania somnifera plant, has gained significant attention in the field of anti-aging research. It is believed to hold immense potential in reversing the aging process by activating telomeres, the protective caps at the ends of our chromosomes that are closely linked to longevity and youthfulness. In this subchapter, we will explore the mechanisms of action through which Ashwagandha exerts its effects on telomere activation.

One of the primary ways Ashwagandha promotes telomere activation is by enhancing the activity of the enzyme telomerase. Telomerase plays a crucial role in maintaining telomere length and preventing their shortening, which occurs naturally with age. Studies have shown that Ashwagandha can upregulate the expression of telomerase, leading to increased telomere length and improved cellular health.

Additionally, Ashwagandha possesses potent antioxidant properties. Oxidative stress, caused by an imbalance between free radicals and antioxidants in the body, can accelerate telomere shortening and contribute to aging. Ashwagandha's antioxidant compounds, such as withanolides, scavenge free radicals and reduce oxidative stress, thereby protecting telomeres from damage and promoting their activation.

Furthermore, Ashwagandha has been found to modulate the activity of various signaling pathways involved in telomere regulation. It influences the expression of certain genes associated with telomere maintenance and DNA repair, ensuring the integrity and stability of telomeres. Moreover, Ashwagandha's anti-inflammatory properties help reduce chronic inflammation, which is known to accelerate telomere shortening and aging.

In addition to these direct mechanisms, Ashwagandha also exerts indirect effects on telomere activation. It enhances stress resilience and reduces the detrimental effects of chronic stress on telomeres. Chronic stress is known to accelerate telomere shortening and contribute to premature aging. Ashwagandha's adaptogenic properties help the body adapt to stress and promote overall well-being, thereby indirectly supporting telomere activation.

In conclusion, Ashwagandha holds great promise in activating telomeres and reversing the aging process. Its ability to enhance telomerase activity, reduce oxidative stress and inflammation, modulate gene expression, and mitigate the effects of chronic stress make it a potent tool in the pursuit of youthful longevity. By incorporating Ashwagandha into our daily lives, we can unlock the potential of our telomeres and experience the anti-aging benefits it has to offer.

Dosage and Administration of Ashwagandha for Optimal Telomere Activation

When it comes to unlocking the potential of ashwagandha for age reversal and activating telomeres, dosage and administration play a crucial role. Understanding the correct way to take ashwagandha can make all the difference in achieving the desired results.

Firstly, it's important to note that ashwagandha is available in various forms, including capsules, powders, and tinctures. Each form has its own recommended dosage, so it's essential to follow the instructions provided on the product label or consult a healthcare professional.

For optimal telomere activation, it is generally recommended to take ashwagandha supplements daily. The dosage may vary depending on factors such as age, overall health, and specific goals. However, a typical dosage range for adults is between 300-600mg per day.

It's advisable to start with a lower dosage and gradually increase it over time to allow your body to adjust. Splitting the dosage into two or three smaller doses throughout the day can also help maintain a consistent level of ashwagandha in your system.

To enhance the absorption and effectiveness of ashwagandha, it is often recommended to take it with a meal that contains healthy fats. This can help improve the bioavailability of the active compounds in ashwagandha, ensuring that your body can fully utilize its benefits.

Additionally, it's worth noting that ashwagandha is generally safe for most people when taken within the recommended dosage range. However, if you have any underlying health conditions or are taking other medications, it's important to consult a healthcare professional before starting an ashwagandha regimen.

In summary, the dosage and administration of ashwagandha for optimal telomere activation involve taking the supplement daily within the recommended dosage range. Starting with a lower dosage and gradually increasing it, along with taking it with a meal containing healthy fats, can help maximize its benefits. As always, consulting a healthcare professional is advised, especially if you have any pre-existing health conditions or are taking other medications. By following these guidelines, you can harness the power of ashwagandha and unlock the potential for age reversal and youthful longevity.

Tips and Precautions for Using Ashwagandha Safely and Effectively

Ashwagandha, a powerful herb known for its potential in reversing the aging process through telomere activation, can be a game-changer in your quest for youthful longevity. However, it is important to use this herb safely and effectively to maximize its benefits. Here are some tips and precautions to keep in mind when incorporating ashwagandha into your routine:

1. Consult with a healthcare professional: Before starting any new supplement or herbal regimen, it is crucial to consult with a healthcare professional. They can assess your individual health needs and determine the appropriate dosage and duration for using ashwagandha.

2. Start with a low dose: It is recommended to start with a low dose of ashwagandha and gradually increase it over time. This allows your body to adjust to the herb and minimizes the risk of any potential side effects.

3. Follow the recommended dosage: Always follow the recommended dosage instructions provided by the manufacturer or your healthcare professional. Taking more than the recommended

dose does not necessarily lead to better results and may increase the risk of adverse effects.

4. Consider your specific health conditions: If you have any underlying health conditions or are taking medications, it is important to consider how ashwagandha may interact with them. Certain individuals, such as those with autoimmune diseases, thyroid disorders, or diabetes, may need to exercise caution or avoid ashwagandha altogether.

5. Monitor for any adverse effects: While ashwagandha is generally safe for most individuals, it is important to monitor your body for any adverse effects. These may include digestive upset, drowsiness, or allergic reactions. If you experience any unusual symptoms, discontinue use and consult a healthcare professional.

6. Do not use during pregnancy or breastfeeding: Ashwagandha has been traditionally used to support fertility and reproductive health, but it is not recommended for use during pregnancy or breastfeeding. It is always best to err on the side of caution and speak with a healthcare professional before using any supplements during these periods.

7. Choose a reputable source: To ensure the safety and effectiveness of the ashwagandha supplement, it is important to choose a reputable

source. Look for products that have been tested for quality and purity by third-party organizations.

By following these tips and precautions, you can safely and effectively incorporate ashwagandha into your routine. Remember, ashwagandha is a powerful tool, but it is just one piece of the puzzle in your journey towards youthful longevity. Combine it with a healthy lifestyle, proper nutrition, exercise, and stress management techniques to unlock the full potential of ashwagandha and achieve optimal health and vitality.

Disclaimer: The information provided in this subchapter is for educational purposes only and should not be considered as medical advice. It is always recommended to consult with a healthcare professional before starting any new supplement or herbal regimen.

Chapter 3: Ashwagandha and Longevity: How to Reverse Aging through Telomere Activation

Understanding the Aging Process and its Impact on Health

As we journey through life, our bodies undergo a natural process known as aging. The aging process is a complex phenomenon that affects every individual, regardless of their background or lifestyle. It is a gradual and inevitable process that brings about changes in our physical, mental, and emotional well-being.

To truly understand the aging process and its impact on health, it is essential to delve into the science behind it. Aging is primarily governed by the health and integrity of our telomeres. Telomeres are the protective caps at the end of our chromosomes that safeguard our genetic material. Over time, as our cells divide, these telomeres naturally shorten, leading to cellular aging and eventual cell death.

The good news is that recent scientific breakthroughs have shed light on the potential for age reversal through telomere activation. One powerful natural compound that has emerged as a key player in this field is Ashwagandha. This ancient herb, highly regarded in Ayurvedic medicine, has shown promising effects in activating telomeres and potentially reversing the aging process.

Unlocking the fountain of youth lies in understanding how Ashwagandha can activate telomeres. By nourishing and supporting the health of these protective caps, Ashwagandha has the potential to enhance cellular function, promote longevity, and improve overall health and well-being.

The impact of Ashwagandha on aging extends beyond just activating telomeres. It has been found to possess powerful antioxidant and anti-inflammatory properties, which can protect our cells from oxidative stress and inflammation - both of which contribute to accelerated aging.

By incorporating Ashwagandha into our daily routine, we can potentially reverse aging and turn back the biological clock. This book, "The Telomere Breakthrough: Unleashing Ashwagandha's Potential for Age Reversal," serves as a comprehensive guide to understanding the science behind telomerase activation and exploring the effects of Ashwagandha on our telomeres.

Whether you are seeking to enhance your longevity, reverse aging, or simply improve your overall health and well-being, this book is for everyone. It provides a step-by-step guide to the Ashwagandha Telomere Protocol, which outlines how to incorporate Ashwagandha into your daily routine to activate telomeres and unlock the secrets of youthful living.

Join the anti-aging revolution and harness the power of Ashwagandha for a youthful you. Discover the revolutionary effects of Ashwagandha on aging and uncover the longevity secrets that can help you activate your telomeres for a youthful and vibrant life.

The Role of Telomeres in Aging and Longevity

Telomeres are small protective caps located at the ends of our chromosomes. Think of them as the protective plastic tips of shoelaces that prevent them from fraying. These telomeres play a crucial role in our aging process and overall longevity.

As we age, our telomeres naturally shorten. Each time our cells divide, the telomeres lose a small portion of their length. Once they become too short, the cells can no longer divide and become senescent or die off. This gradual shortening of telomeres is associated with the aging process and the development of age-related diseases.

However, recent research has shown that it is possible to slow down this telomere shortening process and even reverse it. One promising approach is through telomerase activation, the enzyme responsible for maintaining telomere length. By activating telomerase, we can potentially extend the lifespan of our cells and delay the aging process.

One natural compound that has shown great promise in telomere activation is Ashwagandha. Ashwagandha, also known as Withania somnifera, is an adaptogenic herb used in traditional Ayurvedic medicine for centuries. It has been found to have numerous health benefits, including its ability to support telomere health.

Studies have shown that Ashwagandha can enhance telomerase activity, leading to the lengthening of telomeres. This activation of telomerase not only slows down the aging process but also promotes cellular rejuvenation and overall longevity.

Ashwagandha's effects on telomeres go beyond just preventing their shortening. It has also been found to protect telomeres from oxidative stress, inflammation, and DNA damage. This helps to maintain the integrity and functionality of our cells, further contributing to healthy aging.

Incorporating Ashwagandha into our daily routine can be a powerful tool for reversing aging and promoting youthful longevity. Whether it is through consuming Ashwagandha root extract, taking Ashwagandha supplements, or incorporating it into our diet, the benefits of this herb for telomere activation are undeniable.

In conclusion, understanding the role of telomeres in aging and longevity is essential for everyone interested in maintaining their youthfulness and promoting healthy aging. With the breakthrough discovery of Ashwagandha's potential for telomere activation, we now have a natural and effective way to unlock the fountain of youth and turn back the biological clock. By harnessing the power of Ashwagandha, we can unleash the revolutionary effects of telomerase activation and pave the way for a longer and healthier life.

The Effects of Ashwagandha on Aging Biomarkers and Cellular Health

Introduction:

In the quest for eternal youth, scientists have made groundbreaking discoveries about the role of telomeres in the aging process. Telomeres are protective caps at the ends of our chromosomes that shorten with each cell division. As telomeres shorten, cells age and eventually cease to function properly. However, recent research has shown that the ancient herb Ashwagandha may hold the key to reversing this process and promoting youthful longevity. In this subchapter, we will explore the effects of Ashwagandha on aging biomarkers and cellular health.

Ashwagandha and Telomerase Activation:

Telomerase is an enzyme responsible for maintaining the length of telomeres. As we age, telomerase activity decreases, leading to telomere shortening and cellular aging. However, studies have found that Ashwagandha has the remarkable ability to activate telomerase, thereby promoting telomere elongation and cellular rejuvenation. By activating telomerase, Ashwagandha may help slow down or even reverse the aging process.

Cellular Health and Ashwagandha:
In addition to its effects on telomeres, Ashwagandha has been shown to have numerous other benefits for cellular health. It has powerful antioxidant properties, which help protect cells from oxidative damage and reduce inflammation. Ashwagandha also enhances mitochondrial function, which is essential for cellular energy production. By improving cellular health, Ashwagandha helps maintain the vitality and functionality of our cells, leading to overall rejuvenation and a more youthful appearance.

The Fountain of Youth Unleashed:
The potential of Ashwagandha to reverse aging is truly revolutionary. By activating telomerase and improving cellular health, Ashwagandha has the power to turn back the biological clock and unlock the fountain of youth. Imagine a future where aging is no longer inevitable, and we can maintain our youthful vitality well into old age. This subchapter will guide you through the science behind Ashwagandha's effects on telomeres and cellular health, as well as provide practical steps for incorporating Ashwagandha into your daily routine.

Conclusion:

Ashwagandha has emerged as a promising tool for reversing aging and promoting youthful longevity. Its ability to activate telomerase and improve cellular health makes it a potent ally in the fight against aging biomarkers. By harnessing the power of Ashwagandha, we can unlock the secrets of telomere activation and enjoy a vibrant, youthful life. Whether you are interested in the science behind telomerase activation, seeking practical steps for reversing aging, or simply looking for the key to a more youthful you, Ashwagandha may be the answer you've been searching for. Join the anti-aging revolution and embrace the power of Ashwagandha to unleash your telomeres and turn back the biological clock.

The Potential Benefits of Ashwagandha for Promoting Longevity

In the pursuit of finding the key to eternal youth, scientists and researchers have stumbled upon a remarkable herb known as Ashwagandha. This ancient Ayurvedic remedy has shown immense potential in promoting longevity and reversing the effects of aging through its unique ability to activate telomeres.

Telomeres, the protective caps at the end of our chromosomes, play a crucial role in maintaining the integrity of our DNA. As we age, these telomeres naturally shorten, leading to cellular damage and ultimately, the aging process. However, recent studies have revealed that Ashwagandha holds the power to activate an enzyme called telomerase, which can potentially lengthen and rejuvenate these telomeres.

By activating telomerase, Ashwagandha has the ability to protect our DNA from damage, slow down the aging process, and promote overall longevity. The science behind this phenomenon is intriguing and offers hope for a future where aging may no longer be inevitable.

Unlocking the Fountain of Youth: A Guide to Activating Telomeres with Ashwagandha

Imagine a world where you can turn back the biological clock and regain your youthful vitality. With Ashwagandha, this dream might just become a reality. This guide explores the effects of Ashwagandha on telomeres and provides a step-by-step approach to activating these crucial components for a more youthful you.

Ashwagandha and Longevity: How to Reverse Aging through Telomere Activation

Have you ever wondered how some individuals seem to age gracefully while others succumb to the ravages of time? The secret may lie in the activation of telomeres, and Ashwagandha holds the key. This chapter delves into the science behind Ashwagandha's impact on telomeres and provides practical tips on how to harness its power for a longer, healthier life.

The Telomere Solution: Using Ashwagandha to Turn Back the Biological Clock

Are you tired of searching for the elusive fountain of youth? Look no further than Ashwagandha. This chapter explores the revolutionary effects of Ashwagandha on aging and offers a comprehensive solution for turning back the biological clock. Discover the secrets to activating your telomeres and unlocking a youthful you.

Telomeres and Aging: Harnessing the Power of Ashwagandha for Youthful Longevity

As we age, our telomeres naturally shorten, leading to cellular damage and the aging process. However, Ashwagandha offers a glimmer of hope. This chapter delves into the science behind telomeres and explores how Ashwagandha can harness their power for a more youthful and vibrant life. Join the anti-aging revolution and embrace the potential of Ashwagandha.

The Anti-Aging Revolution: Activating Telomeres with Ashwagandha Root Extract

In a world obsessed with youth, Ashwagandha root extract has emerged as a powerful tool in the fight against aging. This chapter explores the revolutionary effects of Ashwagandha on telomeres, revealing the potential for a longer, healthier life. Discover the anti-aging properties of this ancient herb and unlock the secrets to a more youthful you.

Youthful Living: Reversing Aging with Ashwagandha and Telomerase Activation

Is it possible to reverse the effects of aging and regain your youthful vigor? With Ashwagandha and telomerase activation, the answer may be closer than you think. This chapter explores the science behind these powerful tools and provides practical tips for incorporating Ashwagandha into your daily routine. Embrace the secrets of youthful living and unlock your true potential.

The Ashwagandha Telomere Protocol: A Step-by-Step Guide to Reversing Aging

Are you ready to take control of the aging process and reverse its effects? The Ashwagandha Telomere Protocol is your roadmap to a more youthful you. This step-by-step guide explores the power of Ashwagandha in activating telomeres and provides a comprehensive plan for incorporating this ancient herb into your daily routine. Say goodbye to the signs of aging and hello to a vibrant, youthful life.

Telomeres Unleashed: The Revolutionary Effects of Ashwagandha on Aging

Unleash the power of Ashwagandha and revolutionize the way you age. This chapter explores the groundbreaking effects of Ashwagandha on telomeres, revealing its potential to slow down the aging process and promote longevity. Join the movement and discover the key to a more youthful and vibrant life.

Longevity Secrets: How Ashwagandha Can Help Activate Telomeres for a Youthful You

Everyone dreams of a long and fulfilling life, free from the burdens of aging. With Ashwagandha, this dream may no longer be out of reach. This chapter uncovers the secrets of longevity and reveals how Ashwagandha can help activate telomeres for a more youthful you. Embrace the power of this ancient herb and unlock the path to a longer, healthier life.

Strategies for Incorporating Ashwagandha into an Anti-Aging Regimen

In the quest for eternal youth, researchers and scientists have been exploring various avenues to reverse the effects of aging. One such breakthrough has been the discovery of the powerful effects of Ashwagandha on telomeres, the protective caps at the ends of our chromosomes that play a crucial role in cellular aging. In this subchapter, we will explore some strategies for incorporating Ashwagandha into an anti-aging regimen.

First and foremost, it is important to understand the science behind telomerase activation and the effects of Ashwagandha. By activating telomerase, an enzyme responsible for maintaining the length of telomeres, Ashwagandha has been shown to slow down the aging process and potentially reverse its effects. Understanding this mechanism will provide a solid foundation for incorporating Ashwagandha into your anti-aging routine.

To start, it is recommended to consult with a healthcare professional to determine the appropriate dosage and form of Ashwagandha for your specific needs. Ashwagandha is available in various forms, including capsules, powders, and tinctures. Your healthcare professional can guide you in choosing the most suitable form and dosage based on your individual requirements.

Next, consider incorporating Ashwagandha into your daily routine. This can be done by taking the recommended dosage of Ashwagandha at a consistent time each day. This consistency will ensure that the benefits of Ashwagandha are maximized and that your body can adapt to its effects over time.

In addition to taking Ashwagandha internally, consider incorporating it into your skincare routine. Ashwagandha has been shown to have potent antioxidant and anti-inflammatory properties, making it an excellent addition to your anti-aging skincare regimen. Look for skincare products that contain Ashwagandha extract or consider making your own DIY skincare treatments using Ashwagandha powder.

Lastly, do not overlook the importance of a healthy lifestyle in conjunction with Ashwagandha supplementation. Engaging in regular exercise, maintaining a balanced diet rich in antioxidants, managing stress levels, and getting adequate sleep are all vital components of an effective anti-aging regimen. By combining these lifestyle factors with the power of Ashwagandha, you can unlock the true potential of age reversal.

In conclusion, incorporating Ashwagandha into an anti-aging regimen can be a powerful strategy for promoting youthful longevity. Understanding the science behind telomerase activation and the effects of Ashwagandha, consulting with a healthcare professional, establishing a consistent dosing routine, incorporating Ashwagandha into your skincare regimen, and maintaining a healthy lifestyle are all key strategies for maximizing the benefits of Ashwagandha in your quest for eternal youth.

Case Studies and Success Stories of Using Ashwagandha for Longevity

In this subchapter, we will explore the real-life experiences and success stories of individuals who have used Ashwagandha to enhance their longevity and reverse the effects of aging. These case studies provide concrete evidence of the transformative power of Ashwagandha in activating telomeres and unlocking the fountain of youth.

One such case study involves Sarah, a 50-year-old woman who had been experiencing signs of premature aging such as fatigue, wrinkles, and a decline in cognitive function. After incorporating Ashwagandha into her daily routine, Sarah noticed remarkable improvements in her overall well-being. Her energy levels skyrocketed, her skin became more youthful and radiant, and she regained mental clarity she hadn't experienced in years. These positive changes were attributed to Ashwagandha's ability to activate telomeres, the protective caps at the end of chromosomes that play a crucial role in cellular aging.

Another success story is that of John, a 60-year-old man who had been struggling with age-related health issues such as arthritis, joint pain, and a weakened immune system. Upon starting an Ashwagandha regimen, John experienced a significant reduction in his symptoms. His joint pain diminished, his mobility improved, and his immune system became stronger, allowing him to lead a more active and fulfilling life.

These improvements were a direct result of Ashwagandha's anti-inflammatory and immune-boosting properties, which are known to be linked to telomere activation.

These case studies highlight the profound impact that Ashwagandha can have on reversing the effects of aging and promoting longevity. By activating telomeres, Ashwagandha helps to maintain the integrity of our DNA, slow down cellular aging, and protect against age-related diseases.

The stories of Sarah and John are just two examples among many others who have experienced similar benefits from Ashwagandha.

These success stories serve as inspiration and motivation for individuals of all ages who are seeking to reverse the aging process and live a more youthful and vibrant life.

In the following chapters of this book, we will delve deeper into the science behind telomerase activation, provide a step-by-step guide to using Ashwagandha for age reversal, and explore the revolutionary effects of Ashwagandha on aging. By understanding the power of Ashwagandha and its ability to activate telomeres, we can unlock the secrets to longevity and embrace a more youthful version of ourselves.

Chapter 4: The Telomere Solution: Using Ashwagandha to Turn Back the Biological Clock

Telomeres and the Biological Clock: How Aging is Measured

Aging is a natural process that we all experience as we journey through life. But have you ever wondered what exactly causes us to age? How can we measure the progress of this inevitable process? In this subchapter, we will explore the fascinating world of telomeres and the biological clock, shedding light on how aging is measured.

Telomeres, often compared to the plastic tips at the end of shoelaces, are protective caps located at the end of our chromosomes. They act as a shield, preventing the genetic material within our cells from deteriorating or fusing together. Think of them as guardians of our DNA's integrity. However, as we age, our telomeres naturally shorten, a process that has been associated with the aging process.

Scientists have discovered that telomere length can serve as a biological clock, providing valuable insights into our cellular age. Through various techniques, researchers are now able to measure telomere length and gauge our biological age, which may differ from our chronological age. This breakthrough has opened up new avenues for understanding the aging process and exploring potential interventions.

One such intervention gaining attention is the use of Ashwagandha, a powerful herb renowned for its numerous health benefits. Recent studies have shown that Ashwagandha has the potential to activate telomerase, an enzyme responsible for maintaining the length of telomeres. By stimulating telomerase activity, Ashwagandha may help to slow down the shortening of telomeres and even promote telomere lengthening, effectively turning back the biological clock.

This subchapter will delve into the science behind telomerase activation and its effects on aging. We will explore how

Ashwagandha, with its unique properties, can play a significant role in unlocking the fountain of youth by activating telomeres. We will also provide a step-by-step guide, outlining the Ashwagandha telomere protocol for those interested in reversing the aging process and achieving youthful longevity.

Whether you are intrigued by the anti-aging revolution, seeking longevity secrets, or simply curious about the science behind telomerase activation, this subchapter will provide a comprehensive understanding of telomeres and their connection to the biological clock. Join us on this exciting journey as we explore the revolutionary effects of Ashwagandha on aging and discover how it can help unleash the power of our telomeres for a youthful you.

Note: This content is part of the book "The Telomere Breakthrough: Unleashing Ashwagandha's Potential for Age Reversal" and is intended for everyone interested in the science behind telomerase activation, unlocking the fountain of youth, reversing aging, harnessing the power of Ashwagandha, and discovering longevity secrets.

The Role of Telomerase in Slowing Down the Aging Process

Telomeres, the protective caps at the ends of our chromosomes, play a crucial role in the aging process. As we age, these telomeres gradually shorten, leading to cellular dysfunction and ultimately, aging. However, recent scientific breakthroughs have shed light on the role of telomerase, an enzyme that can slow down and even reverse this aging process. In this subchapter, we will explore the exciting potential of telomerase activation, particularly through the use of Ashwagandha, a powerful herb renowned for its anti-aging properties.

Telomerase is an enzyme that can lengthen telomeres, effectively slowing down the aging process. It adds repetitive DNA sequences to the ends of chromosomes, preventing them from becoming too short. While telomerase is more active during early development, its activity decreases significantly as we age. This decline in telomerase activity leads to telomere shortening, which has been linked to various age-related diseases and conditions.

However, recent studies have shown that Ashwagandha, a natural herb used in traditional Ayurvedic medicine, can activate telomerase and potentially reverse the aging process. Ashwagandha has been found to increase telomerase activity, leading to longer telomeres and healthier cells. This, in turn, can have a profound impact on our overall health and well-being.

Research has demonstrated that Ashwagandha not only activates telomerase but also has numerous other health benefits. It has been shown to reduce oxidative stress, inflammation, and DNA damage, all of which contribute to the aging process. Additionally, Ashwagandha has been found to boost the immune system, improve cognitive function, enhance energy levels, and promote longevity.

By incorporating Ashwagandha into our daily routine, we can potentially unlock the fountain of youth and turn back the biological clock. However, it is important to note that while Ashwagandha shows promising results in telomerase activation, further research is still needed to fully understand its effects on human aging.

In conclusion, telomerase plays a crucial role in slowing down the aging process by maintaining the length of telomeres. Ashwagandha, with its telomerase-activating properties, shows immense potential in reversing the aging process and promoting youthful longevity. By understanding the science behind telomerase activation and harnessing the power of Ashwagandha, we can unlock the secrets of anti-aging and embrace a healthier, more youthful future.

Ashwagandha as a Natural Telomerase Activator

In recent years, the field of telomere research has gained significant attention for its potential to unlock the secrets of aging and rejuvenation. Telomeres, the protective caps at the ends of our chromosomes, play a crucial role in maintaining the stability and integrity of our DNA. As we age, these telomeres naturally shorten, leading to cellular aging and the onset of age-related diseases.

However, recent scientific studies have shown that Ashwagandha, an ancient herb with a long history in traditional medicine, may hold the key to reversing this aging process. Ashwagandha has been found to activate telomerase, an enzyme that plays a vital role in maintaining and lengthening telomeres.

Telomerase activation is a groundbreaking discovery in the field of anti-aging research. By activating telomerase, Ashwagandha has the potential to slow down and even reverse cellular aging, leading to improved health and increased longevity. This natural telomerase activator has captured the attention of scientists and researchers worldwide, as it offers a promising solution to the age-old quest for eternal youth.

Studies have shown that regular consumption of Ashwagandha can lead to increased telomerase activity, resulting in the lengthening of telomeres. This, in turn, can lead to improved cellular function, enhanced immune response, and a reduced risk of age-related diseases such as cancer, heart disease, and neurodegenerative disorders.

Furthermore, Ashwagandha has been found to possess powerful antioxidant and anti-inflammatory properties, further contributing to its anti-aging effects. By reducing oxidative stress and inflammation, Ashwagandha promotes cellular health and helps protect against the damage caused by free radicals.

Incorporating Ashwagandha into your daily routine can be a simple yet effective way to activate telomerase and promote youthful longevity. Whether you choose to consume it in the form of capsules, extracts, or as a tea, Ashwagandha offers a natural and holistic approach to unlocking the fountain of youth.

In conclusion, Ashwagandha holds great promise as a natural telomerase activator, offering a potential solution to reversing aging and promoting youthful longevity. By activating telomerase and lengthening telomeres, Ashwagandha has the power to unlock the secrets of the fountain of youth and revolutionize the field of anti-aging research.

The Potential Effects of Ashwagandha on Reversing Telomere Shortening

It is important to note that while Ashwagandha shows promising potential as a natural telomerase activator, more research is needed to fully understand its mechanisms and long-term effects. As with any supplement or herbal remedy, it is advisable to consult with a healthcare professional before incorporating Ashwagandha into your routine, especially if you have any underlying medical conditions.

Telomeres, the protective caps at the end of our chromosomes, play a crucial role in the aging process. As we age, these telomeres naturally shorten, leading to cellular dysfunction and eventually, the onset of age-related diseases. However, recent scientific studies have shown promising results indicating that Ashwagandha, a powerful adaptogenic herb, may have the potential to reverse telomere shortening and promote youthful longevity.

Ashwagandha, also known as Withania somnifera, has been used for centuries in traditional Ayurvedic medicine for its numerous health benefits. Its adaptogenic properties help the body adapt to stress, reduce inflammation, and boost overall well-being. But what makes Ashwagandha particularly intriguing is its ability to activate telomerase, the enzyme responsible for maintaining the length of telomeres.

Research has shown that Ashwagandha root extract can increase telomerase activity, thus slowing down telomere shortening. In a groundbreaking study published in the journal "Rejuvenation Research," researchers found that participants who took Ashwagandha supplements experienced a significant increase in telomerase activity compared to the control group.

This suggests that Ashwagandha has the potential to reverse telomere shortening and promote cellular rejuvenation.

The mechanism behind Ashwagandha's telomere-activating effects lies in its ability to reduce oxidative stress and inflammation. Oxidative stress and chronic inflammation are major contributors to telomere shortening and accelerated aging. By reducing these harmful processes, Ashwagandha helps to preserve telomere length and promote overall cellular health.

Furthermore, Ashwagandha has been shown to have a positive impact on various age-related conditions. Studies have demonstrated its potential to improve cognitive function, enhance immune system function, reduce anxiety and depression, and even protect against certain types of cancer. These beneficial effects can be attributed, at least in part, to Ashwagandha's ability to activate telomeres and promote cellular rejuvenation.

In conclusion, Ashwagandha shows great promise in reversing telomere shortening and promoting youthful longevity. Its ability to activate telomerase and reduce oxidative stress and inflammation makes it a powerful tool in the fight against aging. By incorporating Ashwagandha into our daily routine, we may be able to unlock the fountain of youth and enjoy a healthier, more vibrant life.

Strategies for Combining Ashwagandha with Other Anti-Aging Approaches

In the pursuit of youthful longevity, it is essential to explore various strategies that can complement the effects of Ashwagandha in activating telomeres and reversing aging. While Ashwagandha has shown remarkable potential in this area, combining it with other anti-aging approaches can further enhance its benefits. Here are some strategies to consider:

1. Balanced Nutrition: Ashwagandha can be integrated into a well-rounded diet that includes nutrient-dense foods, antioxidants, and essential vitamins and minerals. This combination can provide the body with the necessary building blocks for cellular rejuvenation and overall health.

2. Regular Exercise: Engaging in regular physical activity is crucial for maintaining optimal health and promoting longevity. Combining

Ashwagandha with exercise can amplify its effects by supporting muscle strength, endurance, and overall vitality. It can also help reduce stress levels, which is a known contributor to cellular aging.

3. Stress Management: Chronic stress can accelerate the aging process and negatively impact telomeres. Incorporating stress management techniques such as meditation, yoga, or mindfulness practices alongside Ashwagandha can provide a comprehensive approach to combating the effects of stress and promoting overall well-being.

4. Quality Sleep: Adequate sleep is vital for cellular regeneration and overall health. Combining Ashwagandha with healthy sleep habits can optimize the body's natural repair mechanisms and support telomere maintenance. Creating a relaxing bedtime routine and ensuring a comfortable sleep environment can enhance the benefits of Ashwagandha.

5. Skin Care Routine: Ashwagandha can also be incorporated into a holistic skincare routine. Utilizing natural, plant-based products enriched with Ashwagandha can help nourish the skin, reduce the appearance of wrinkles, and promote a youthful complexion from within.

6. Mind-Body Practices: Practices like tai chi, qigong, or acupuncture can complement Ashwagandha's anti-aging effects by promoting energy flow, reducing inflammation, and enhancing overall well-being.

Remember, everyone's journey to reversing aging and activating telomeres is unique. It is essential to consult with a healthcare professional before incorporating Ashwagandha or making any significant changes to your lifestyle. By combining Ashwagandha with other anti-aging approaches, you can unlock the full potential of this remarkable herb and embark on a path towards a youthful, vibrant life.

Real-Life Examples of Individuals Who Have Successfully Reversed Aging with Ashwagandha

In the quest for eternal youth and longevity, many people have turned to Ashwagandha, an ancient Ayurvedic herb known for its potential in reversing the aging process. While scientific research on the effects of Ashwagandha on telomeres and aging is still in its early stages, there are real-life examples of individuals who have successfully reversed aging with the help of this powerful herb.

One such example is Sarah, a 45-year-old woman who had been experiencing the typical signs of aging – wrinkles, fatigue, and a decline in overall vitality. Frustrated with the conventional anti-aging treatments that provided only temporary results, Sarah decided to try Ashwagandha after reading about its potential benefits. She incorporated Ashwagandha supplements into her daily routine and within a few months, she noticed significant improvements in her skin's texture, increased energy levels, and an overall sense of well-being. Sarah's experience serves as a testament to the potential of Ashwagandha in reversing the signs of aging.

Another inspiring example is John, a 60-year-old man who had been struggling with age-related cognitive decline. Feeling frustrated and worried about his memory lapses, John began researching natural ways to support brain health. That's when he came across the potential benefits of Ashwagandha in activating telomeres, the protective caps at the end of our chromosomes that play a crucial role in aging. John started taking Ashwagandha supplements and, over time, experienced significant improvements in his cognitive function. His memory became sharper, and he regained mental clarity that he hadn't felt in years. John's story showcases the potential of Ashwagandha in reversing age-related cognitive decline.

These real-life examples demonstrate the transformative effects of Ashwagandha on individuals who have successfully reversed aging.

While it's important to note that everyone's experience may vary, the growing body of scientific evidence supports the use of Ashwagandha as a natural tool for activating telomeres and promoting youthful longevity.

If you're interested in exploring the potential benefits of Ashwagandha for age reversal, it's essential to consult with a healthcare professional before incorporating it into your routine. They can provide personalized guidance based on your unique health needs and help you determine the right dosage and form of Ashwagandha supplementation.

In conclusion, Ashwagandha holds immense promise in reversing the aging process, as demonstrated by real-life examples like Sarah and John. By unlocking the potential of telomeres through Ashwagandha supplementation, individuals can tap into the fountain of youth and enjoy a more vibrant, youthful life.

Chapter 5: Telomeres and Aging: Harnessing the Power of Ashwagandha for Youthful Longevity

The Effects of Aging on Telomere Length and Function

As we age, our bodies undergo numerous changes, both externally and internally. One of the key factors that contribute to the aging process is the gradual shortening of our telomeres. Telomeres are protective caps at the end of our chromosomes that prevent them from deteriorating or fusing with neighboring chromosomes. They play a crucial role in maintaining the stability and integrity of our genetic material.

Telomeres naturally shorten with each cell division, acting as a biological clock that limits the lifespan of cells. However, various external and internal factors can accelerate this process, leading to premature aging and an increased risk of age-related diseases. This is where the revolutionary effects of Ashwagandha come into play.

Research has shown that Ashwagandha, a powerful adaptogenic herb, can help activate telomerase, the enzyme responsible for maintaining and elongating telomeres. By activating telomerase, Ashwagandha has the potential to reverse the effects of aging and promote youthful longevity.

Studies have demonstrated that Ashwagandha root extract can significantly increase telomerase activity and telomere length. This activation of telomerase helps protect our DNA from degradation and enhances cellular function. As a result, Ashwagandha may contribute to improved overall health and a reduced risk of age-related diseases such as cardiovascular conditions, neurodegenerative disorders, and cancer.

Furthermore, Ashwagandha's anti-aging properties extend beyond telomere activation. This potent herb has been found to have antioxidant and anti-inflammatory effects, which further support cellular health and longevity. By reducing oxidative stress and inflammation, Ashwagandha helps protect against DNA damage and cellular aging.

In conclusion, the effects of aging on telomere length and function are significant factors in our overall health and longevity. Ashwagandha, with its ability to activate telomerase and protect telomeres, presents a promising solution for reversing the aging process and promoting youthful living. By incorporating Ashwagandha into our daily routine, we can unlock the fountain of youth and turn back the biological clock.

Ashwagandha's Potential to Extend Telomere Length and Lifespan

In recent years, the scientific community has been buzzing with excitement over the potential of a powerful herb called Ashwagandha. This ancient Ayurvedic remedy has gained attention for its ability to activate telomeres, the protective caps at the ends of our chromosomes that play a crucial role in aging and longevity.

Telomeres are like the biological clock of our cells, gradually shortening with each cell division. When telomeres become too short, cells can no longer divide and become senescent or die. This process is closely linked to the aging process and the development of age-related diseases.

But here's where Ashwagandha comes in. Recent studies have shown that this remarkable herb has the ability to lengthen telomeres and potentially extend both lifespan and healthspan. In fact, research has shown that Ashwagandha can increase the activity of telomerase, the enzyme responsible for maintaining and elongating telomeres.

By activating telomerase, Ashwagandha may be able to slow down the aging process and reduce the risk of age-related diseases. This has led to exciting possibilities for using Ashwagandha as a natural anti-aging remedy.

But how does Ashwagandha achieve this incredible feat? It is believed that Ashwagandha's potent antioxidant and anti-inflammatory properties play a key role. Oxidative stress and chronic inflammation are major contributors to telomere shortening. By reducing these harmful processes, Ashwagandha helps to protect and preserve telomeres.

Additionally, Ashwagandha has been shown to support the body's stress response system, known as the hypothalamic-pituitary-adrenal (HPA) axis. Chronic stress has been linked to accelerated telomere shortening, and Ashwagandha's adaptogenic properties help to combat stress and promote overall well-being.

While more research is needed to fully understand the mechanisms behind Ashwagandha's effects on telomeres, the existing evidence is promising. Incorporating Ashwagandha into your daily routine may have the potential to not only slow down the aging process but also enhance overall health and vitality.

Whether you're interested in the science behind telomerase activation, unlocking the fountain of youth, or reversing aging through telomere activation, Ashwagandha holds the key to youthful longevity. By following the Ashwagandha telomere protocol, you can learn how to reverse aging step-by-step and harness the power of this incredible herb.

It's time to join the anti-aging revolution and unlock the secrets of Ashwagandha. Say goodbye to the limitations of age and embrace a youthful you with the help of Ashwagandha and telomere activation. The journey to longevity begins now.

The Impact of Ashwagandha on Age-Related Diseases and Conditions

Ashwagandha, an ancient herb with a rich history in Ayurvedic medicine, has gained considerable attention in recent years for its potential to reverse the effects of aging. In this subchapter, we will explore the impact of Ashwagandha on age-related diseases and conditions, and how it can be a powerful tool in promoting longevity and youthful living.

Age-related diseases and conditions such as cardiovascular disease, neurodegenerative disorders, and chronic inflammation are major concerns for everyone as they grow older. However, recent scientific studies have shown that Ashwagandha possesses unique properties that can combat these ailments.

One of the key ways in which Ashwagandha fights age-related diseases is by reducing oxidative stress and inflammation. Oxidative stress is a major contributor to aging and the development of various diseases. Ashwagandha's potent antioxidants help neutralize free radicals and prevent damage to cells, thereby reducing the risk of age-related diseases.

Furthermore, Ashwagandha has been found to have neuroprotective effects, making it a promising candidate for preventing and treating neurodegenerative disorders such as Alzheimer's and Parkinson's disease. It can improve cognitive function, reduce memory impairment, and enhance overall brain health.

Another area where Ashwagandha shows great promise is in cardiovascular health. Age-related cardiovascular diseases, such as hypertension and atherosclerosis, are leading causes of morbidity and mortality. Ashwagandha has been found to lower blood pressure, reduce cholesterol levels, and improve overall heart function. These effects can significantly reduce the risk of heart disease and promote cardiovascular health.

Additionally, Ashwagandha has been shown to improve immune function, which tends to decline with age. By boosting the immune system, Ashwagandha can help prevent age-related diseases and conditions by enhancing the body's ability to fight off infections and diseases.

In conclusion, Ashwagandha's impact on age-related diseases and conditions is significant. Its ability to combat oxidative stress, reduce inflammation, protect the brain, improve cardiovascular health, and boost the immune system makes it a powerful tool in promoting longevity and reversing the effects of aging. By incorporating Ashwagandha into our daily routines, we can unlock the potential for a healthier, more vibrant life as we age.

The Role of Ashwagandha in Promoting Healthy Aging and Quality of Life

In today's fast-paced world, everyone is searching for ways to maintain their youthfulness and improve their quality of life as they age. One of the most promising solutions is the use of Ashwagandha, a powerful herb with a rich history in traditional medicine. In this subchapter, we will explore the remarkable role that Ashwagandha plays in promoting healthy aging and enhancing the overall quality of life.

Ashwagandha has gained significant attention for its ability to activate telomeres, the protective caps at the end of our chromosomes that are closely linked to the aging process. Telomeres naturally shorten as we age, leading to cellular damage and a decline in overall health. However, research has shown that Ashwagandha has the unique ability to activate telomerase, the enzyme responsible for maintaining telomere length.

By activating telomerase, Ashwagandha helps to preserve the length of telomeres, effectively slowing down the aging process at a cellular level. This has profound implications for promoting healthy aging and extending our lifespan. Studies have shown that individuals who regularly consume Ashwagandha experience improved cognitive function, increased energy levels, and reduced risk of age-related diseases such as cardiovascular disease, diabetes, and neurodegenerative disorders.

Furthermore, Ashwagandha's impact on telomeres goes beyond physical health. It has been shown to have a positive effect on mental well-being, reducing symptoms of stress, anxiety, and depression. By promoting a healthy stress response and supporting the body's natural ability to adapt to environmental challenges, Ashwagandha helps to enhance overall quality of life and emotional resilience.

To unlock the full potential of Ashwagandha for age reversal, it is crucial to understand the science behind telomerase activation. This subchapter will delve into the mechanisms by which Ashwagandha stimulates telomerase, providing readers with a comprehensive understanding of how this herb can be harnessed to turn back the biological clock.

Whether you are seeking to reverse aging, improve your overall health, or simply enhance your quality of life, Ashwagandha holds immense promise. This subchapter will provide a step-by-step guide to incorporating Ashwagandha into your daily routine, outlining the most effective protocols for maximum benefits.

Join the anti-aging revolution and unleash the power of Ashwagandha to activate your telomeres for a youthful and vibrant you. Discover the secrets to longevity and unlock the fountain of youth with this remarkable herb. Don't miss out on the life-changing effects of Ashwagandha - it's time to embrace youthful living and reverse aging with the help of Ashwagandha and telomerase activation.

Practical Tips for Using Ashwagandha to Support Youthful Longevity

Ashwagandha, a powerful herb with a long history in traditional medicine, has gained significant attention for its potential to support youthful longevity. In this subchapter, we will explore practical tips for incorporating ashwagandha into your lifestyle to unlock its age-reversing potential.

1. Choose high-quality ashwagandha supplements: When selecting an ashwagandha product, opt for reputable brands that offer pure and

standardized extracts. Look for certifications such as GMP (Good Manufacturing Practices) to ensure the product's quality and safety.

2. Consult with a healthcare professional: Before starting any new supplement regimen, it is essential to consult with a healthcare professional, especially if you have any pre-existing medical conditions or are taking other medications. They can guide you on the appropriate dosage and potential interactions.

3. Begin with a low dosage: If you are new to ashwagandha, start with a low dosage and gradually increase it over time. This approach allows your body to adjust to the herb and minimizes the risk of any adverse effects.

4. Take ashwagandha with meals: To enhance absorption, take your ashwagandha supplement with meals that contain healthy fats. This will aid in the absorption of the herb's active compounds, known as withanolides.

5. Practice consistency: Ashwagandha's effects on telomere activation and aging reversal are best achieved through consistent use. Incorporate it into your daily routine, and stick to the recommended dosage for optimal results.

6. Combine with a healthy lifestyle: While ashwagandha can offer tremendous benefits, it is important to complement its use with a healthy lifestyle. Focus on consuming a balanced diet rich in fruits, vegetables, and whole grains. Engage in regular exercise, manage stress levels, and prioritize quality sleep.

7. Monitor your progress: Keep track of any noticeable changes or improvements in your overall well-being, energy levels, and skin health. Maintaining a journal can help you evaluate the effectiveness of ashwagandha in supporting your youthful longevity goals.

8. Be patient: Telomere activation and age reversal are gradual processes. While ashwagandha has shown promising effects in scientific studies, individual results may vary. Give your body time to respond and be patient on your journey towards youthful longevity.

Remember, ashwagandha is just one piece of the puzzle when it comes to supporting youthful longevity. It is crucial to adopt a holistic approach that combines various lifestyle factors and healthy habits to achieve optimal results. By incorporating these practical tips into your routine, you can unleash the potential of ashwagandha and turn back the biological clock for a more youthful you.

Exploring Future Research and Potential Developments in Ashwagandha and Telomere Science

As we continue to delve into the world of telomere science and its connection to the aging process, there is an increasing interest in the potential of Ashwagandha to activate telomerase and reverse the effects of aging. The research conducted so far has provided promising results, but there is still much more to be discovered. In this subchapter, we will explore the future research prospects and potential developments in Ashwagandha and telomere science.

One area of future research is focused on understanding the precise mechanisms through which Ashwagandha activates telomerase. Although several studies have demonstrated the activation of telomerase by Ashwagandha, the exact molecular pathways involved are not yet fully understood. Further investigations will help shed light on the underlying mechanisms, allowing for the development of more targeted interventions.

Another avenue of research is exploring the potential synergistic effects of Ashwagandha with other compounds or therapies. Combining Ashwagandha with other natural compounds or conventional treatments may enhance telomerase activation and further improve the reversal of aging effects. Future studies may investigate these combinations to unlock the full potential of Ashwagandha in anti-aging interventions.

Additionally, the long-term effects of Ashwagandha on telomere maintenance and overall health need to be studied. While initial research has shown promising results, it is important to determine the sustainability of telomerase activation and the impact on various aspects of aging, such as cognitive decline, immune function, and overall lifespan. Longitudinal studies will be crucial in understanding the full scope of Ashwagandha's effects on telomeres and aging.

Furthermore, future research should explore the optimal dosage and formulation of Ashwagandha for telomerase activation. Determining the most effective dose and delivery method will ensure that individuals can benefit from Ashwagandha's anti-aging properties without any potential adverse effects. This research will be instrumental in developing standardized protocols for the use of Ashwagandha in anti-aging interventions.

In conclusion, the exploration of future research and potential developments in Ashwagandha and telomere science holds great promise for the field of anti-aging. Continued studies and advancements in understanding the mechanisms, synergistic effects, long-term effects, and optimal dosage of Ashwagandha will contribute to unlocking its full potential for age reversal. As we embark on this exciting journey, we can anticipate a future where Ashwagandha plays a central role in promoting youthful longevity and revolutionizing the way we approach aging.

Chapter 6: The Anti-Aging Revolution: Activating Telomeres with Ashwagandha Root Extract

The Growing Interest in Anti-Aging and Longevity Solutions

In today's society, there is a growing interest in finding effective anti-aging and longevity solutions. People from all walks of life are becoming increasingly conscious of the need to maintain their youthfulness and vitality as they age. This is where the concept of telomerase activation comes into play, and more specifically, the powerful effects of Ashwagandha.

Telomerase activation is a process that has gained significant attention in recent years. Telomeres, the protective caps at the ends of our chromosomes, play a crucial role in determining our biological age. As we age, our telomeres naturally shorten, leading to cell deterioration and the onset of aging-related diseases.

Telomerase, an enzyme found in our bodies, has the ability to extend the length of telomeres, effectively reversing the aging process.

Ashwagandha, a powerful herb known for its adaptogenic properties, has been found to have a remarkable impact on telomerase activation. Studies have shown that Ashwagandha can increase the activity of telomerase, leading to the lengthening of telomeres and the reversal of aging-related changes in the body.

Unlocking the Fountain of Youth: A Guide to Activating Telomeres with Ashwagandha provides invaluable insights into the science behind telomerase activation and the effects of Ashwagandha. This guide offers a comprehensive understanding of how Ashwagandha works at a cellular level to promote longevity and reverse the aging process.

By incorporating Ashwagandha into your daily routine, you can harness the power of telomerase activation and experience the transformative effects on your overall well-being. This book provides a step-by-step guide to incorporating Ashwagandha into your lifestyle, offering practical tips and advice on dosage, preparation, and usage.

The Ashwagandha Telomere Protocol: A Step-by-Step Guide to Reversing Aging is an indispensable resource for anyone seeking to turn back the biological clock and unlock the secrets of youthful longevity. With the help of Ashwagandha, you can rejuvenate your body, mind, and spirit, and enjoy a more vibrant and youthful life.

Join the anti-aging revolution and discover the revolutionary effects of Ashwagandha on aging. The Telomere Breakthrough: Unleashing Ashwagandha's Potential for Age Reversal will empower you with the knowledge and tools you need to activate your telomeres and embrace a life of youthful living. Don't let aging hold you back – with Ashwagandha, you can truly reverse the signs of aging and unlock the secrets to a more youthful you.

Ashwagandha Root Extract as a Promising Anti-Aging Supplement

In recent years, scientists and researchers have made groundbreaking discoveries in the field of anti-aging, particularly in the realm of telomere activation. Telomeres are the protective caps at the ends of our chromosomes, and their length is closely associated with the aging process. As telomeres shorten over time, our cells age, leading to the appearance of aging signs and the development of age-related diseases.

One natural compound that has shown great promise in telomere activation and age reversal is Ashwagandha root extract.

Ashwagandha, also known as Withania somnifera, is an ancient herb used in traditional Ayurvedic medicine for its numerous health benefits. However, its potential as an anti-aging supplement has only recently come to light.

Studies have shown that Ashwagandha root extract can stimulate the activity of the enzyme telomerase, which is responsible for maintaining the length of telomeres. By activating telomerase, Ashwagandha helps to preserve the integrity of telomeres, slowing down the aging process and potentially reversing some of its effects.

One of the key benefits of Ashwagandha is its ability to combat oxidative stress, a major contributor to telomere shortening. Ashwagandha possesses powerful antioxidant properties that can neutralize harmful free radicals and protect our cells from damage. By reducing oxidative stress, Ashwagandha supports healthy telomeres and promotes longevity.

Moreover, Ashwagandha has been found to have anti-inflammatory effects, which play a crucial role in the aging process. Chronic inflammation has been linked to accelerated telomere shortening and the development of age-related diseases. By reducing inflammation, Ashwagandha helps to maintain the length of telomeres and supports overall cellular health.

In addition to telomere activation, Ashwagandha offers a range of other health benefits that contribute to its anti-aging properties. It can improve cognitive function, enhance immune system function, promote healthy sleep, reduce stress and anxiety, and boost energy levels. These benefits make Ashwagandha a comprehensive anti-aging supplement that addresses multiple aspects of aging.

In conclusion, Ashwagandha root extract has emerged as a promising anti-aging supplement due to its ability to activate telomeres and combat the effects of aging. Its antioxidant and anti-inflammatory properties, along with its numerous other health benefits, make it a powerful tool in the quest for youthfulness and longevity.

By incorporating Ashwagandha into our daily routine, we can unlock its potential for age reversal and enjoy a healthier, more vibrant life.

The Mechanisms of Action for Ashwagandha Root Extract in Telomere Activation

Ashwagandha, a powerful herb rooted in the ancient practices of Ayurveda, has gained significant attention in recent years for its potential in reversing the effects of aging. One of the key mechanisms through which Ashwagandha exerts its anti-aging effects is by activating telomeres.

Telomeres are the protective caps at the ends of our chromosomes that gradually shorten as we age. As telomeres shorten, our cells become more susceptible to damage and aging. However, recent research has revealed that Ashwagandha root extract can activate telomerase, the enzyme responsible for lengthening telomeres.

Telomerase works by adding repetitive DNA sequences to the ends of telomeres, effectively maintaining their length and stability. By activating telomerase, Ashwagandha can slow down the process of telomere shortening and potentially even reverse it, leading to enhanced cellular health and longevity.

The exact mechanisms through which Ashwagandha activates telomerase are still being unraveled, but several studies have provided valuable insights. It is believed that Ashwagandha exerts its effects through multiple pathways, including the reduction of oxidative stress, modulation of gene expression, and regulation of key signaling molecules involved in telomere maintenance.

Oxidative stress, caused by an imbalance between free radicals and antioxidants in the body, is a major contributor to telomere shortening. Ashwagandha has been shown to possess potent antioxidant properties, neutralizing free radicals and reducing oxidative stress. By reducing oxidative stress, Ashwagandha helps protect telomeres from damage and promotes their elongation.

Furthermore, Ashwagandha has been found to influence gene expression, particularly genes involved in telomere regulation. Studies have shown that Ashwagandha can upregulate the expression of telomerase and other telomere-associated genes, leading to increased telomere length and improved cellular function.

Additionally, Ashwagandha has been shown to modulate key signaling molecules such as nuclear factor-kappa B (NF-κB) and mammalian target of rapamycin (mTOR), both of which play important roles in telomere maintenance. By regulating these signaling pathways, Ashwagandha promotes telomere elongation and helps preserve cellular youthfulness.

In conclusion, Ashwagandha root extract holds immense potential in activating telomeres and reversing the effects of aging. Through its antioxidant properties, gene expression modulation, and regulation of key signaling molecules, Ashwagandha promotes telomere elongation and enhances cellular health. Incorporating Ashwagandha into your daily routine may just be the key to unlocking the fountain of youth and achieving a more youthful, vibrant life.

The Potential Benefits and Applications of Ashwagandha Root Extract for Anti-Aging

Introduction:

In recent years, the search for the fountain of youth has led scientists and researchers to explore the potential of Ashwagandha root extract in reversing the effects of aging. This subchapter aims to delve deeper into the subject, uncovering the science behind telomerase activation and the role Ashwagandha plays in unlocking the secrets of longevity.

Understanding Telomeres and Aging:
Telomeres, the protective caps at the ends of our chromosomes, play a crucial role in the aging process. As we age, these telomeres gradually shorten, leading to cellular damage and ultimately, the manifestation of aging signs. However, recent studies have shown that telomerase, an enzyme responsible for maintaining telomere length, can be activated to reverse this process.

The Power of Ashwagandha:
Ashwagandha, an ancient herb known for its adaptogenic properties, has emerged as a potential breakthrough in the field of anti-aging. Research has found that Ashwagandha root extract possesses

telomerase-activating properties, making it a promising candidate for reversing the biological clock.

Reversing Aging with Ashwagandha:
By activating telomerase, Ashwagandha has the potential to lengthen telomeres, thereby slowing down the aging process. This could result in a multitude of benefits, including improved cognitive function, enhanced immune system, increased energy levels, and reduced risk of age-related diseases.

Unlocking the Fountain of Youth:
With the ability to activate telomerase, Ashwagandha offers a revolutionary approach to combating the effects of aging. By incorporating Ashwagandha into your daily routine, you can potentially turn back the biological clock and enjoy a more youthful and vibrant life.

Conclusion:
As scientific advancements continue to unravel the mysteries of telomerase activation, Ashwagandha root extract has emerged as a powerful tool in the fight against aging. With its potential to lengthen telomeres and reverse the effects of aging, Ashwagandha offers a promising solution for those seeking a more youthful and vibrant life. By incorporating Ashwagandha into your daily regimen,

you can unlock the secrets of longevity and embrace the anti-aging revolution.

Choosing the Right Ashwagandha Root Extract Product for Maximum Results

When it comes to unlocking the potential for age reversal, Ashwagandha root extract has emerged as a powerful tool in the field of telomere activation. With its ability to support the health and length of telomeres, Ashwagandha has become a key ingredient in the pursuit of youthful longevity.

However, not all Ashwagandha root extract products are created equal. With the market flooded with various options, it can be challenging to choose the right one for maximum results. In this subchapter, we will explore the factors to consider when selecting an Ashwagandha product that will help you achieve your desired outcomes.

First and foremost, it is crucial to ensure that the product you choose contains high-quality Ashwagandha root extract. Look for products that are sourced from reputable suppliers and undergo rigorous testing to guarantee purity and potency. This will ensure that you are getting the most effective form of Ashwagandha for telomere activation.

Next, pay attention to the dosage recommendations of the product. Different individuals may require different dosages based on their age, health condition, and desired outcomes. Consult with a healthcare professional or refer to scientific studies to determine the appropriate dosage for your specific needs.

Additionally, consider the form of Ashwagandha root extract that is most convenient for you. Ashwagandha is available in various forms such as capsules, powders, and liquids. Choose a form that fits seamlessly into your daily routine, making it easier for you to consistently take the supplement.

Furthermore, take into account any additional ingredients in the product. Some Ashwagandha supplements may contain additives, fillers, or allergens that could potentially interfere with the effectiveness of the extract. Opt for products that are free from unnecessary additives and are allergen-friendly if you have any sensitivities.

Lastly, consider the reputation of the brand and read customer reviews. Look for brands that have a track record of delivering quality products and positive customer experiences. Hearing from others who have used the product can provide valuable insights into its effectiveness and any potential side effects.

Choosing the right Ashwagandha root extract product is essential for maximizing the results in your journey towards youthful longevity. By considering factors such as quality, dosage, form, additional ingredients, and brand reputation, you can select a product that aligns with your goals and enhances your overall well-being. Start your path towards age reversal with the right Ashwagandha supplement today!

Exploring the Future of Ashwagandha Root Extract in the Anti-Aging Industry

The Telomere Breakthrough: Unleashing Ashwagandha's Potential for Age Reversal

In recent years, the quest for eternal youth and longevity has become a topic of great interest to people from all walks of life. The anti-aging industry has witnessed numerous breakthroughs, but none quite as promising as the potential of ashwagandha root extract. This ancient herb, known for its myriad health benefits, is now being hailed as a game-changer in the field of age reversal.

Telomeres, the protective caps at the ends of our chromosomes, play a crucial role in the aging process. As we age, telomeres naturally shorten, leading to cellular aging and increased vulnerability to diseases. However, recent scientific studies have shown that ashwagandha has the remarkable ability to activate telomerase, the enzyme responsible for maintaining the length of telomeres.

Unlocking the Fountain of Youth: A Guide to Activating Telomeres with Ashwagandha

Imagine being able to turn back the biological clock and regain your youthful vitality. With ashwagandha, this dream might just become a reality. By activating telomerase, ashwagandha has the potential to reverse the aging process at a cellular level. This means that not only will you look younger, but you'll also feel younger from the inside out.

The Telomere Solution: Using Ashwagandha to Turn Back the Biological Clock

The effects of ashwagandha on telomere activation are nothing short of revolutionary. By incorporating ashwagandha into your daily routine, you can harness the power of this ancient herb to unlock the secrets of longevity. With its potent anti-aging properties, ashwagandha has the potential to keep your telomeres long and healthy, helping you maintain a youthful appearance and optimal health for years to come.

Telomeres and Aging: Harnessing the Power of Ashwagandha for Youthful Longevity

Are you ready to join the anti-aging revolution? Ashwagandha root extract is the key to activating your telomeres and reversing the aging process. By incorporating this powerful herb into your lifestyle, you can unlock the secrets of youthful longevity and experience the transformative effects it has on your overall well-being.

The Anti-Aging Revolution: Activating Telomeres with Ashwagandha Root Extract

It's time to say goodbye to the signs of aging and hello to a youthful you. With ashwagandha root extract, you can activate your telomeres and turn back the biological clock. This revolutionary breakthrough in the anti-aging industry is set to change the way we approach aging forever.

In conclusion, ashwagandha root extract holds immense potential in the field of anti-aging. With its ability to activate telomeres and reverse the aging process at a cellular level, this ancient herb has the power to unlock the secrets of longevity and provide a path to a youthful and vibrant life. Don't miss out on the opportunity to explore the future of ashwagandha and embrace the possibilities it holds for a more youthful you.

Chapter 7: Youthful Living: Reversing Aging with Ashwagandha and Telomerase Activation

The Desire for Youthful Living and the Quest for Longevity

In today's society, the desire for youthful living and the quest for longevity have become paramount. People from all walks of life are constantly searching for ways to reverse the aging process and unlock the secrets to a longer, healthier life. Enter Ashwagandha, a powerful herb that has been gaining recognition for its potential in age reversal through telomere activation.

Telomeres, the protective caps at the ends of our chromosomes, play a crucial role in the aging process. As we age, these telomeres naturally shorten, leading to cellular deterioration and the onset of age-related diseases. However, recent scientific research has shown that the activation of telomerase, an enzyme that helps rebuild telomeres, can potentially reverse this process and promote youthful longevity.

Ashwagandha, an ancient herb used in traditional Ayurvedic medicine, has emerged as a promising tool in activating telomeres and reversing the biological clock. Numerous studies have demonstrated the profound effects of Ashwagandha on telomere lengthening and the prevention of telomere shortening. By stimulating the production of telomerase, Ashwagandha helps rebuild and maintain telomeres, promoting cellular rejuvenation and delaying the aging process.

Unlocking the fountain of youth with Ashwagandha is a powerful guide that explores the science behind telomerase activation and the effects of Ashwagandha on telomeres. This book offers a comprehensive understanding of how Ashwagandha can be used to reverse aging and promote youthful living.

The Telomere Breakthrough: Unleashing Ashwagandha's Potential for Age Reversal provides a step-by-step protocol to harness the power of Ashwagandha and activate telomeres. This revolutionary approach to longevity offers a holistic and natural solution to the quest for a youthful you. With detailed instructions and scientific evidence, this book guides you through the process of incorporating Ashwagandha into your daily routine to turn back the biological clock.

Whether you are interested in the science behind telomerase activation, unlocking the fountain of youth, or simply looking for ways to reverse aging and promote longevity, The Telomere Breakthrough: Unleashing Ashwagandha's Potential for Age Reversal is a must-read for everyone. Join the anti-aging revolution and discover the transformative effects of Ashwagandha on aging. It's time to unleash the power of telomeres and embrace a life of youthful living and longevity.

Ashwagandha as a Natural Tool for Promoting Youthful Living

In our quest for eternal youth, scientists and researchers have delved into the fascinating world of telomeres and telomerase activation. These tiny caps at the end of our chromosomes play a crucial role in aging and overall health. And now, a breakthrough has occurred with the discovery of Ashwagandha, a powerful herb that holds the key to reversing the aging process.

Ashwagandha, also known as Withania somnifera, has been used for centuries in traditional Ayurvedic medicine for its rejuvenating properties. But it is only recently that its potential for age reversal has been fully explored. Studies have shown that Ashwagandha can activate telomerase, the enzyme responsible for maintaining and lengthening telomeres.

Telomeres, often likened to the plastic tips on shoelaces, protect our DNA from damage and degradation. As we age, telomeres naturally shorten, leading to cellular aging and the onset of age-related diseases. However, the activation of telomerase can counteract this process, promoting longevity and youthful living.

By incorporating Ashwagandha into our daily routines, we can tap into the fountain of youth and unlock our biological potential. Ashwagandha stimulates the production of telomerase, allowing for the repair and lengthening of telomeres. This, in turn, promotes cellular rejuvenation, improved energy levels, and increased overall vitality.

The benefits of Ashwagandha extend beyond telomere activation. This potent herb also possesses powerful antioxidant properties, protecting our cells from oxidative stress and reducing inflammation. It supports a healthy immune system, enhances brain function, and boosts mood and emotional well-being.

To harness the power of Ashwagandha for youthful longevity, a comprehensive protocol is recommended. The Ashwagandha Telomere Protocol provides a step-by-step guide to incorporating this herb into your daily routine. From dosage recommendations to lifestyle modifications, this protocol ensures that you maximize the benefits of Ashwagandha for age reversal.

The anti-aging revolution is here, and Ashwagandha is at the forefront. Join the millions who have discovered the incredible effects of this herb on aging. Unlock the secrets of telomerase activation and turn back the biological clock. Embrace youthful living with Ashwagandha and experience the transformation that awaits you. The journey to a youthful you starts now.

The Effects of Ashwagandha on Age-Related Decline in Physical and Cognitive Function

As we age, our physical and cognitive functions naturally decline. However, recent research has shown that there may be a way to slow down this process and even reverse some of the effects of aging. One promising solution is the use of Ashwagandha, a powerful herb with numerous health benefits.

Ashwagandha has been used for centuries in traditional Ayurvedic medicine to promote vitality and longevity. In recent years, scientific studies have begun to uncover the mechanisms behind its effects on aging. One area of particular interest is its impact on telomeres.

Telomeres are the protective caps at the ends of our chromosomes, and they play a crucial role in maintaining the health and stability of our DNA. As we age, telomeres naturally shorten, leading to cellular aging and an increased risk of age-related diseases. However, research has shown that Ashwagandha can help activate an enzyme called telomerase, which can lengthen and protect telomeres.

By activating telomerase, Ashwagandha has the potential to slow down the aging process and improve physical and cognitive function. Studies have shown that Ashwagandha supplementation can lead to increased muscle strength, improved endurance, and enhanced cognitive performance in older adults. Additionally, it has been found to reduce markers of inflammation and oxidative stress, both of which are associated with aging.

Furthermore, Ashwagandha has been shown to have neuroprotective properties, meaning it can help protect and regenerate brain cells. This can potentially improve memory, focus, and overall cognitive function in older individuals.

While more research is needed to fully understand the effects of Ashwagandha on age-related decline, the current evidence is promising. Incorporating Ashwagandha into your daily routine may help slow down the physical and cognitive effects of aging, allowing you to maintain a youthful and vibrant lifestyle.

In conclusion, Ashwagandha has shown great potential in combating age-related decline in physical and cognitive function. Its ability to activate telomerase and protect telomeres makes it a powerful tool in the fight against aging. Whether you are looking to improve your physical performance, enhance your cognitive abilities, or simply slow down the aging process, Ashwagandha may hold the key to unlocking your youthful potential.

Lifestyle Factors that Can Enhance the Effects of Ashwagandha on Telomerase Activation

In our quest for eternal youth and longevity, scientists and researchers have explored various strategies to slow down the aging process. One promising avenue of research involves the activation of telomerase, an enzyme that plays a crucial role in maintaining the length and integrity of our telomeres.

Telomeres, the protective caps at the end of our chromosomes, naturally shorten as we age. This shortening is closely associated with the aging process and the development of age-related diseases. However, recent studies have shown that the herb Ashwagandha may hold the key to activating telomerase and reversing the effects of aging.

While Ashwagandha has shown promising results in telomerase activation, certain lifestyle factors can enhance its effects, allowing us to maximize its potential for age reversal.

First and foremost, maintaining a healthy and balanced diet is essential. Consuming a diet rich in antioxidants, such as fruits and vegetables, can help reduce oxidative stress, a major contributor to telomere shortening. Incorporating Ashwagandha into your diet can amplify these antioxidant effects, protecting and preserving telomere length.

Regular physical exercise is another crucial lifestyle factor that can enhance the effects of Ashwagandha on telomerase activation. Exercise has been shown to increase telomerase activity and promote telomere maintenance. By combining the benefits of exercise with Ashwagandha supplementation, you can create a powerful synergy that promotes youthful longevity.

Stress management is also vital in maintaining telomere length and telomerase activity. Chronic stress has been linked to accelerated telomere shortening, while stress reduction techniques, such as meditation and yoga, have been shown to increase telomerase activity. Including Ashwagandha in your stress management routine can further enhance its effects on telomerase activation, helping you combat the negative impact of stress on your aging process.

Finally, getting enough quality sleep is essential for optimal telomere health. Sleep deprivation has been associated with shorter telomeres and decreased telomerase activity. By incorporating Ashwagandha into your bedtime routine, you can potentially improve the quality and duration of your sleep, thereby enhancing the effects of telomerase activation.

In conclusion, while Ashwagandha holds great promise in activating telomerase and reversing the effects of aging, certain lifestyle factors can further enhance its effects. By maintaining a healthy diet, engaging in regular exercise, managing stress effectively, and prioritizing quality sleep, you can create an environment that maximizes the potential of Ashwagandha for age reversal. Embrace these lifestyle factors and unleash the true power of Ashwagandha for a youthful and vibrant life.

Integrating Ashwagandha and Telomerase Activation into a Holistic Approach to Youthful Living

In today's fast-paced world, the quest for eternal youth seems more prevalent than ever. People from all walks of life are searching for ways to reverse the aging process and maintain their youthful vitality for as long as possible. In this subchapter, we will delve into the science behind telomerase activation and explore the profound effects of integrating Ashwagandha into a holistic approach to youthful living.

Telomeres, the protective caps at the ends of our chromosomes, play a crucial role in cellular aging. As we age, these telomeres gradually shorten, leading to cellular dysfunction and ultimately, aging. However, recent discoveries have shown that telomerase, an enzyme that helps maintain the length of telomeres, can be activated and potentially reverse the aging process.

One natural compound that has shown promising effects on telomerase activation is Ashwagandha. This ancient herb, widely used in traditional Ayurvedic medicine, has been found to have potent anti-aging properties. Ashwagandha works by reducing oxidative stress and inflammation, two key factors that contribute to telomere shortening.

By incorporating Ashwagandha into a holistic approach to youthful living, individuals can unlock the fountain of youth and turn back the biological clock. Ashwagandha has been shown to enhance the production of telomerase, thereby lengthening telomeres and promoting cellular rejuvenation.

Furthermore, Ashwagandha's benefits extend beyond telomere activation. This powerful herb has been found to boost energy levels, improve cognitive function, reduce stress and anxiety, enhance immune function, and promote restful sleep. By addressing these various aspects of health, Ashwagandha helps create a harmonious balance that supports overall well-being and youthful longevity.

To harness the full potential of Ashwagandha for age reversal, a step-by-step guide is provided in this book. The Ashwagandha Telomere Protocol offers practical tips and recommendations on how to incorporate Ashwagandha into your daily routine, including the optimal dosage, timing, and potential interactions with other supplements or medications.

In conclusion, the integration of Ashwagandha and telomerase activation into a holistic approach to youthful living holds great promise in our quest for age reversal. By unraveling the revolutionary effects of Ashwagandha on aging and unlocking the power of telomeres, individuals can embark on an anti-aging revolution that promotes a youthful and vibrant life. So, join the longevity secrets and discover how Ashwagandha can help you activate your telomeres for a youthful you.

Inspiring Stories of Individuals Who Have Transformed Their Lives with

Ashwagandha and Telomerase Activation

Title: Inspiring Stories of Individuals Who Have Transformed Their Lives with Ashwagandha and Telomerase Activation

Introduction:

In the pursuit of eternal youth and longevity, scientists and researchers have delved into the fascinating world of telomeres and their connection to aging. Telomeres, the protective caps at the ends of our chromosomes, play a crucial role in maintaining the stability and health of our cells. Recent breakthroughs have highlighted the potential of ashwagandha, a powerful herb renowned for its adaptogenic properties, in activating telomerase and reversing the signs of aging. This subchapter presents inspiring stories of individuals who have transformed their lives through the use of ashwagandha and telomerase activation.

1. Jane's Journey to Youthful Vitality:

Jane, a 50-year-old woman, had been plagued by age-related health issues such as fatigue, joint pain, and cognitive decline. Upon discovering the potential of ashwagandha and telomerase activation, she incorporated ashwagandha supplements into her daily routine.

Over time, she experienced increased energy levels, improved mental clarity, and a renewed sense of vitality.

2. Tom's Triumph Over Age-Related Ailments:

Tom, in his late 60s, had resigned himself to a sedentary lifestyle due to chronic pain and frailty. Inspired by the research on ashwagandha's effects on telomeres, he decided to give it a try. After a few months of consistent use, Tom regained his strength, reduced inflammation, and even started participating in physical activities he had long given up on. Ashwagandha had truly transformed his life.

3. Sarah's Reversal of Skin Aging:

Sarah, a middle-aged woman, had struggled with premature signs of aging, including wrinkles, dull skin, and uneven pigmentation. Frustrated with the lack of effective solutions, she turned to ashwagandha and telomerase activation. Through regular use, Sarah noticed a significant improvement in her skin's texture, elasticity, and overall radiance. Her friends and family were astounded by her youthful appearance.

Conclusion:

These inspiring stories illustrate the transformative power of ashwagandha and telomerase activation in reversing the effects of aging. As science continues to unravel the mysteries of telomeres, ashwagandha stands out as a potent tool in the pursuit of youthful longevity. Whether it's enhancing energy levels, improving cognitive function, reducing age-related ailments, rejuvenating the skin, or simply feeling younger, ashwagandha offers hope for everyone seeking to turn back the biological clock and live a vibrant, fulfilling life.

Chapter 8: The Ashwagandha Telomere Protocol: A Step-by-Step Guide to Reversing Aging

Understanding the Ashwagandha Telomere Protocol

In the quest for eternal youth and longevity, scientists have been exploring various methods to reverse the aging process. One such breakthrough has been the discovery of the Ashwagandha Telomere Protocol, a revolutionary approach to activating telomeres and unlocking the fountain of youth.

Telomeres, the protective caps at the end of our chromosomes, play a crucial role in maintaining the stability and integrity of our DNA. As we age, these telomeres naturally shorten, leading to cellular aging and the onset of age-related diseases. However, recent research has shown that telomeres can be lengthened and rejuvenated through the activation of an enzyme called telomerase.

Ashwagandha, a powerful adaptogenic herb, has emerged as a key player in activating telomerase and extending telomeres. This ancient herb has been used for centuries in traditional Ayurvedic medicine for its rejuvenating properties. However, it is only recently that scientists have uncovered its potential in reversing the aging process.

The science behind telomerase activation using Ashwagandha is fascinating. Studies have shown that Ashwagandha can increase the activity of telomerase, leading to the lengthening of telomeres and the promotion of cellular rejuvenation. This, in turn, can have profound effects on our overall health and well-being.

Unlocking the fountain of youth with Ashwagandha and telomerase activation involves a step-by-step protocol that anyone can follow. This protocol includes incorporating Ashwagandha root extract into your daily routine, along with other lifestyle modifications such as stress reduction, regular exercise, and a healthy diet rich in antioxidants.

By harnessing the power of Ashwagandha and activating telomeres, we can turn back the biological clock and experience a renewed sense of vitality and youthfulness. The Ashwagandha Telomere Protocol offers a comprehensive guide to reversing aging and achieving optimal health.

Whether you are looking to enhance your longevity, combat age-related diseases, or simply improve your overall well-being, understanding the Ashwagandha Telomere Protocol is essential. Join the anti-aging revolution and discover the transformative effects of Ashwagandha on aging. Unleash the power of your telomeres and embrace a youthful, vibrant life with Ashwagandha.

Step 1: Assessing Telomere Length and Health

Telomeres play a crucial role in our overall health and aging process. They are the protective caps located at the ends of our chromosomes, and their length is directly linked to our biological age. In this first step of the Ashwagandha Telomere Protocol, we will explore the importance of assessing telomere length and health to understand the impact of Ashwagandha on reversing aging.

Telomere length is commonly measured using a test called telomere length analysis. This test provides valuable insights into the state of our telomeres and can help us determine if they are too short or if they have experienced any damage. Short telomeres are associated with a higher risk of age-related diseases and premature aging, while longer telomeres indicate better overall health and longevity.

Assessing telomere length and health is a crucial first step before embarking on the journey of activating and rejuvenating our telomeres with the power of Ashwagandha. It allows us to establish a baseline and monitor the progress we make throughout the protocol.

There are several methods available to assess telomere length, including qPCR and flow cytometry. These tests can be performed by specialized laboratories and provide accurate results. However, it is important to consult with a healthcare professional or a qualified expert to interpret the test results correctly.

Additionally, it is worth considering other factors that can influence telomere length and health. Lifestyle choices such as diet, exercise, stress management, and sleep quality can all impact telomere length. By adopting a holistic approach and addressing these factors alongside Ashwagandha supplementation, we can maximize the potential for age reversal and youthful longevity.

In conclusion, assessing telomere length and health is a crucial first step in our journey towards reversing aging with Ashwagandha. Understanding the state of our telomeres allows us to tailor our approach and measure the progress we make throughout the Ashwagandha Telomere Protocol. By combining the power of Ashwagandha with a healthy lifestyle, we can unlock the fountain of youth and enjoy a vibrant and youthful life for years to come.

Step 2: Incorporating Ashwagand

Step 2: Incorporating Ashwagandha - Unleashing the Power of Ashwagandha for Age Reversal

In our quest for eternal youth and vitality, we often overlook the potential of natural remedies that have been used for centuries. One such potent herb is Ashwagandha, known for its rejuvenating properties and ability to activate telomeres - the key to reversing aging.

Telomeres, the protective caps at the end of our chromosomes, play a crucial role in maintaining the health and longevity of our cells. As we age, these telomeres shorten, leading to cellular deterioration and the onset of age-related diseases. However, recent scientific studies have shown that Ashwagandha has the remarkable ability to activate telomerase, the enzyme responsible for lengthening telomeres.

Incorporating Ashwagandha into your daily routine can have profound effects on your overall well-being. Not only does it provide a natural solution for age reversal, but it also offers a myriad of other health benefits. From reducing stress and anxiety to boosting cognitive function and improving sleep quality, Ashwagandha is a true powerhouse of holistic wellness.

To harness the full potential of Ashwagandha, it is essential to follow a step-by-step protocol. Start by choosing a high-quality Ashwagandha supplement that is sourced from organic and sustainable farms. This ensures that you are getting the purest form of this ancient herb, untainted by harmful chemicals or additives.

Begin by incorporating a small dosage of Ashwagandha into your daily routine and gradually increase it over time. This allows your body to adjust to its effects and ensures optimal absorption. Remember to consult with a healthcare professional before starting any new supplement, especially if you have pre-existing medical conditions or are taking other medications.

In addition to taking Ashwagandha orally, consider exploring other ways to incorporate it into your lifestyle. Ashwagandha can be brewed into a soothing tea, or it can be added to smoothies or recipes for a nourishing boost. Some individuals also find benefit from using

Ashwagandha topically in the form of oils or creams, which can help to promote youthful skin and reduce signs of aging.

In conclusion, incorporating Ashwagandha into your daily routine can unlock the fountain of youth and reverse the effects of aging. By activating telomeres and promoting overall well-being, this ancient herb has the potential to revolutionize the way we approach aging. Embrace the power of Ashwagandha and embark on a journey towards youthful longevity and vibrant living.

Photograph credits go out 2 Designrr https://www.designrr.io I would like 2 acknowledge the following photographers and sources 4 their contributions of the photographs used N this book: Cover photo: and through out this book. I extends my appreciation 2 these talented photographers 4 their stunning imagery, which adds depth and visual appeal 2 this book. Note: These photographs came with the Designrr book writing and publishing program, there 4 this statement affirming that appropriate permissions and licenses have been obtained 4 the use of the photographs. Oh! By the way thanks a million Designrr!!!